THE MEDICAL LIBRARIES
OF BOSTON

A Report

READ AT THE FIRST ANNUAL MEETING OF THE BOSTON MEDICAL LIBRARY ASSOCIATION, HELD ON OCTOBER 3, 1876

BY

JAMES R. CHADWICK, M. D.
Librarian of the Association

CAMBRIDGE
Printed at the Riverside Press
1876

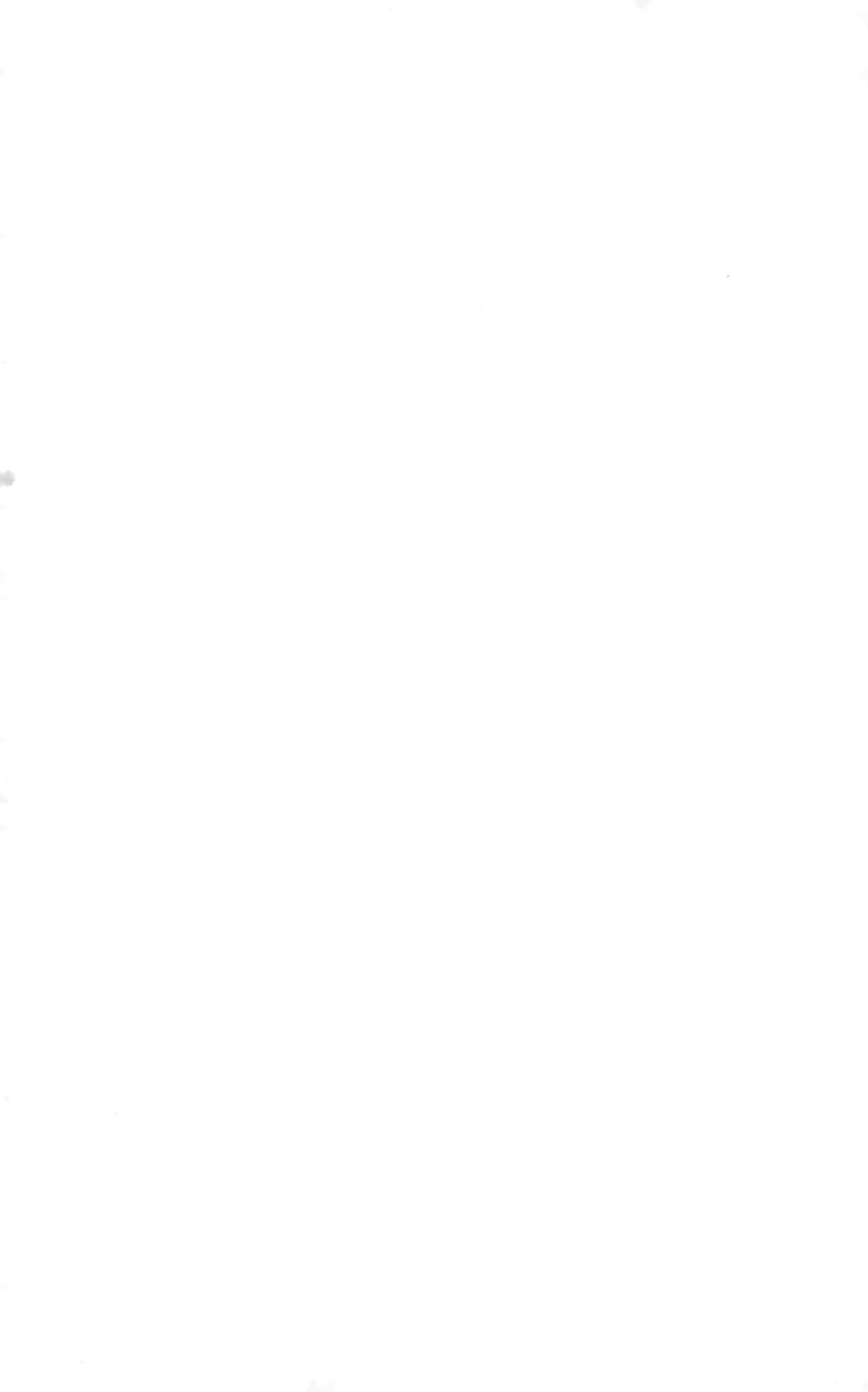

THE MEDICAL LIBRARIES OF BOSTON.

Before entering upon the true domain of this report I propose to pass in brief review the other collections of medical books that have existed in this city, or are held now by various institutions, for the purpose of allowing a few comparisons to be drawn between them and our own library at the end of its first year of existence.

It is gratifying at the outset to learn that our association has adopted the name of almost the first extensive collection of medical books that was made in the city. It would be doubly pleasing could we spread a paternal wing over the books themselves.

THE SECOND SOCIAL OR BOSTON MEDICAL LIBRARY.

In the year of our Lord 1805, Drs. John C. Warren and James Jackson formed a private medical society for mutual improvement, in conjunction with Drs. Dixwell, Coffin, Bullard, Shattuck, Jeffries, Fleet, and Homans. The society came together once a week for the purpose of reading and listening to papers. The members continued to meet until death removed all in succession. From this society, and principally from the exertions of Drs. Warren and Jackson, sprang the Boston Medical Library.[1]

Among the papers of the late Dr. John Jeffries was the following autograph announcement: —

"*December* 30, 1805.

"The Boston Medical Library will be opened on Thursday next at Dr. Fleet's.

"A few books only have arrived.

"N. B. Books received and delivered on Mondays and Thursdays between three and five o'clock, P. M."

[1] Life of John Collins Warren, M. D. By Edward Warren. Vol. i., page 77.

Dr. John Fleet, Jr., lived in Milk Street, and was, I presume, the first librarian.

About the year 1807 the library was entrusted to the care of a sub-librarian, Mr. Amos Smith, apothecary, and "kept in his shop," No. 39 Marlborough Street. The Marlborough Street of those days was the portion of what is now Washington Street which is included between Milk and Bedford streets. The list[1] of books, printed at the time of removal, contains twenty-nine titles and forty-three volumes.

The annual assessment was ten dollars.

In 1826 the Boston Medical Library ceded its whole collection of books, which in 1823 numbered 1311 volumes and was valued at the time of transfer at $4500, to the Athenæum on the following terms: —

It was agreed: "That each proprietor of the medical library should have the privilege of a life-subscriber on the payment of five dollars per annum, and should become a proprietor of the Athenæum by paying one hundred and fifty dollars, such life-subscriber to have the right, on his removal from Boston, to transfer his share for and during the period of his life; that the members of the medical library should have access to the privileges of the Athenæum during the then coming year for the sum of ten dollars; and that the medical department should receive its full proportion of the sums applied hereafter to the purchase of books."

As the shares of the Athenæum were then valued at three hundred dollars, it is probable that nearly all the members of the medical library availed themselves of the opportunity of purchasing at half-price. I find that thirty shares were so taken.

In the letter of Dr. Shattuck dated 1828, which was recently published in the proceedings of the Suffolk District Medical Society,[2] we are in-

[1] I have seen this through the courtesy of Dr. B. J. Jeffries.

[2] Boston Medical and Surgical Journal, September 7, 1876.

formed that there were at that time but seventy-one "regularly-bred" physicians in the city of Boston, so that at least one half of the whole number must have been members of the library. There were only thirty-five physicians who, in his opinion, could support themselves by their practice.

THE ATHENÆUM,

enriched by the above collection, has added to its medical department until it numbers to-day about five thousand volumes. The average annual accessions for the last few years amount to forty volumes, including bound journals. It subscribes to seven American journals, two English, and one French, and to the reports of five London hospitals. Its sets of journals are not numerous, and are notably incomplete.

THE TREADWELL LIBRARY,

at the Massachusetts General Hospital, was founded through the munificence of Dr. J. G. Treadwell, of Salem, in bequeathing, at his death in 1857, to the hospital his own medical library and the sum of forty thousand dollars, of which five thousand dollars were set aside as a permanent fund, the interest of which should be devoted to the purchase of books.[1] This library numbered 3527 volumes on January 1, 1876, and is increasing at the annual rate of about fifty volumes, including the journals, when bound, of which it receives thirty-two regularly. A written catalogue was made in 1860, and has been kept up to date. The library contains full sets of the best English and American journals, but is especially rich in works relating to surgery. The use of the books is restricted to the immediate staff of the hospital, but is accorded to other professional men on written application being made.

1 This library was first offered to the President and Fellows of Harvard College, who declined to accept the bequest on account of the "unusual and embarrassing conditions. What they were I have been unable to discover.

THE HARVARD UNIVERSITY LIBRARY,

in Gore Hall, Cambridge, now contains 3783 medical books. This department of the library was founded by Ward Nicholas Boylston, Esq., who in the year 1802 gave to the college a medical library of eleven hundred volumes, as a special tribute of respect to his uncle, Dr. Zabdiel Boylston. In 1803 he established a permanent fund of five hundred dollars, subsequently augmented, the interest of which was to be expended in the purchase of books and the publication of prize dissertations.

About five hundred volumes were added to this collection a few years since by Dr. B. J. Jeffries, from the library of the late Dr. John Jeffries.

The library contains but few modern works, and hardly any recent periodicals. It receives but one strictly medical journal, and that gratuitously.

THE LIBRARY OF THE HARVARD MEDICAL SCHOOL

consists almost exclusively of old text-books and sets of journals; it is used chiefly by the students of the school, for whom it was avowedly designed by its founders. It originated in a donation of books drawn from the private libraries of the medical faculty in 1819. The number of books may be estimated at about eighteen hundred, of which many are duplicates.

Within a week the physiological laboratory of the medical school has been the recipient of a very large cabinet of microscopic specimens and three hundred and fifty volumes from Dr. John Dean, of this city. The library contains full sets of all the best German, French, and English periodicals relating to anatomy, physiology, and microscopy.

THE BOSTON CITY LIBRARY

has in its medical department, according to the annual report for 1876, 9535 volumes. The average annual increase for the past ten years has been 549 volumes. It receives regularly twenty-four American journals, nineteen English, fourteen French, ten German, and about twenty transactions of societies, making a total of eighty-seven periodicals.

Its collection of journals is very valuable, and the sets are tolerably complete. The trustees are very liberal in purchasing any books desired by the patrons of the institution. The regulations necessitated in a large general library do not allow of access to the shelves except as a special favor. Since the foundation of this library in 1852 many private collections of books have been deposited in its medical alcoves, among others a large portion of the library of the late Dr. James Jackson, and quite recently the library of Dr. D. T. Coit, when he retired from practice. The library of the Massachusetts Medical Society was likewise given to the city a few years ago, at a time when all hope that the profession would ever have a library of its own was entirely relinquished.

This is unquestionably both the largest and the most valuable medical library in the city.

THE BOSTON SOCIETY OF NATURAL HISTORY

has a very choice library of twelve thousand volumes, and receives regularly over five hundred journals, reports, society transactions, etc. Among them are series of all the best journals relating to anatomy, physiology, microscopy, chemistry, botany, and other kindred branches of medical science. Free use of the books is accorded to all who apply for the privilege.

THE BOSTON MEDICAL LIBRARY ASSOCIATION.

It will be manifestly impossible for me to give in detail the individual sources from which the present library has been drawn, or the special character and size of the varied contributions. I shall, however, in this first report, seek to indicate the principal collections of books that the library has received, and make brief acknowledgment to its most prominent benefactors.

The importance of having a reading-room provided with current medical journals and of forming the nucleus of a future medical library of reference, in a locality easy of access from all parts of the city, has long been felt by the profession of Boston. The movement which culminated one year ago in the formation of the present association emanated from the Society for Medical Observation.

The first meeting of six gentlemen at the house of Dr. H. I. Bowditch on December 21, 1874, for the purpose of discussing schemes for a library, was succeeded by others, with a steadily increasing number of participants, during the spring of 1875, and later by a general call to the profession to meet on August 20, 1875. On this occasion organization was effected and officers for the first year were elected.

After a long search the rooms at No. 5 Hamilton Place were secured as possessing the prime requisites of central position and freedom from the noise of passing traffic and of business within doors.

The first extensive collection of books received was that of the Society for Medical Observation, amounting to 911 volumes of the most valuable American, English, French, and German journals. This still constitutes the most useful portion of our library. By the terms of the contract the Observation Society retains full ownership in its library and book-cases, and the right to take from the rooms its own books for the period of one week. It binds its own journals and insures its own library, as heretofore.

The next considerable acquisition of books was the obstetrical library of Dr. William Read, numbering nearly two hundred volumes, and containing nearly all the standard publications on midwifery that have appeared in England during the past century, including many rare and choice works. This department of our library has since been enriched from many other sources, so that it now numbers nearly four hundred titles.

In January, 1876, we received from the trustees of the Boston Dispensary the library left in their building by the late Dr. John Alley. Among other books a large number of the publications of the Sydenham Society were thus added to our resources.

On April 17, 1876, the Boston Society for Medical Improvement deposited its library of 474 volumes in our rooms on the same terms as were accorded to the other society. By this act we acquired many sets of old English and American journals of great rarity and of practical as well as historic worth.

The list of individual contributors is too long to be cited here, yet I cannot pass on without acknowledging the receipt of many volumes bearing the autographs of men whom, I trust, we shall never cease to revere as the leaders of medical thought in New England during the first half of this century: John C. Hayden, George B. Doane, William Ingalls, John Homans, Winslow Lewis, James Jackson, John C. Warren, John Ware, and Charles Gordon. I regard the gifts of these volumes as special testimonials of confidence and encouragement to our infantile institution on the part of the descendants of these worthies.

To David Clapp and Son we are indebted for 271 bound volumes of American and foreign journals, ceded to us for a nominal sum, they being the exchanges of the Boston Medical and Surgical Journal during a portion of the half-century of its publication by that firm.

From these and other contributors, and by exchanges with libraries and individuals in all parts of the country, have been gathered the books that now fill our shelves.

More important, however, than sources of supply and methods of procuring are the results; and I will now render account of the trust that you have reposed in me in a precise statement of the present condition of your collection. The library contains

1339	volumes	of American journals.
739	"	" English "
300	"	" French "
222	"	" German "
23	"	" Canadian "
10	"	" Danish, Norwegian, and Russian journals.
6	"	" Italian and Portuguese journals.

Making a total of

2639	volumes	of journals.
404	"	in the obstetrical section.
1445	"	in general library.
4488	"	in whole library.

I take pleasure in announcing that negotiations are now pending with the Statistical Society which, it is hoped, may result in the deposit of its library of vital statistics in our care. It contains about six hundred volumes of official reports, journals, documents, etc., bearing upon sanitary and vital science, which would prove of great value to all of us who are engaged in researches of this nature.

Of pamphlets we have about three thousand.

To turn now to another distinct purpose of the association, that of providing a reading-room well stocked with current medical literature, I am able to report that we are regularly in receipt of one hundred and twenty medical journals, for twenty-three of which we subscribe, and for the remainder are indebted to the editors and publishers of the Boston Medical and Surgical Journal, who now send us all their exchanges within about one week of the time of their receipt; to the Harvard Medical School, and to Messrs. Codman and Shurtleff, who make over to us all the journals which they respectively receive in consequence of advertisements; and to several individual members of the association who deposit temporarily journals for which they subscribe. From the editors of the North American Review we receive all the medical and scientific books which are sent to them.

It is hoped that our resources may in the coming year allow us to enlarge the list of journals by the addition of some foreign ones that rarely come to this country.

From the treasurer's report you have learned that one hundred and thirty-three members have paid the annual assessment of ten dollars. From the sum thus acquired we have been able to pay our current expenses and one half the cost of furnishing. The residue of indebtedness has been defrayed by the voluntary contributions of many friends, so that we have the gratification of entering upon our second year with a library of four thousand five hundred volumes and three thousand pamphlets, *free from debt.* With a view of extending the facilities of the library and reading-room to the greatest possible number of subscribers, the executive committee have presented the amendment to the by-laws, that you have just voted, reducing the annual fee to six dollars.

A card catalogue with cross references was commenced early in the summer, and is now approaching completion, owing to the indefatigable labors of Drs. E. Wigglesworth, F. H. Brown, E. M. Buckingham, and others.

I cannot close this report without testifying to the prudence of the nominating committee, to the active coöperation of the executive committee, and especially to the deep interest and untiring exertions of your assistant librarian.

Let us enter upon the new year with a firm determination to fulfill the kindly prediction contained in the following paragraph quoted from the highest authority in such matters: "The medical library of most promise in Boston is that of the Medical Library Association, which, though only one year old, has about three thousand volumes, and will probably rapidly increase."[1] Our library already exceeds the figures here adduced by fifteen hundred volumes.

[1] Literature and Institutions, by Dr. J. S. Billings, in The American Journal of the Medical Sciences for October, 1876.